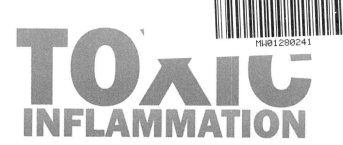

TO*XIC*
INFLAMMATION

WHY YOU'RE TIRED, SICK, AND OVERWEIGHT AND HOW TO BECOME ENERGETIC, HEALTHY, AND FIT!

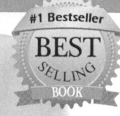

#1 Bestseller
BEST
SELLING
BOOK

CHANCE HAUGEN

Toxic Inflammation

Why You're Tired, Sick, and
Overweight and How to Become
Energetic, Healthy, and Fit!

By Chance Haugen

http://www.inflammationdetox.com/getfreevideos
http://www.chancehaugen.com

Endorsements

So few doctors today go after the root cause of disease. Most doctors are prescribing medications that only cover the symptoms, and alternative doctors give supplements without ever considering the upstream cause. Inflammation is at the root of most diseases, but few ask what is driving the inflammation. Dr. Haugen is one of the few doctors who not only understands that addressing cellular inflammation is the key to modern day illnesses, but goes up stream further and addresses the cause of the cellular inflammation. He believes as do I, that if you don't remove the interference the body will never get well, and even the best supplements money can buy will act only as crutches.

This book offers what so many books on health do not, and that is a real solution. I have said for years "if you don't fix the cell you will never get well" and this book goes to the cell and targets not just inflammation but cellular inflammation "the hidden epidemic". In a toxic world with a growing number of neurotoxins in our food supply and personal lives, cellular inflammation is the new frontier in health care. A growing number of new studies show how these toxins enter our cells causing inflammation and even changing the way our genes express themselves. The inflammation driven by toxins turns on genes for thyroid conditions, weight loss resistance, diabetes and even unexplainable illness represented by fatigue, brain fog and sleep problems. Practitioners like Dr. Haugen who understand this new science in cellular healing are the true answer for the growing number of illnesses that are given no solutions outside the next medication or supplement.

-Dr. Daniel Pompa, D.PSc.

Dr. Chance provides fantastic practical information on the true source of inflammation, which is the cause to disease in America. I recommend everyone to read this book, including doctors. It is very easy to get caught up in dealing with symptoms rather than the true source of people's health issues.

-Dr. Jay Davidson
Founder of Max Health Radio

Dr. Chance Haugen's unique ability to effectively communicate about the "Silent Killer" inflammation in his book Toxic Inflammation, makes it not only a must read for health enthusiasts, but by those who may not know why they do not feel well and have no answers. If you are looking for true answers for your health challenges and are sick and tired of being sick and tired, give Toxic Inflammation a chance to solve your health challenges naturally and safely.

-Warren Phillips M.S.
 Founder Revelation Health LLC

This book is a must read for everyone! Dr. Chance brings to light the damaging effects of inflammation and explains it in ways that anyone can understand. Dr. Chance also gets to the root cause of symptoms and disease, and where the solutions to improving our health lie. This book contains answers to the most common health problems and gives you the ability to take action on your health.

Dr. Meghan Birt
Founder of Just Enjoy Health

Forward

By the founder of LifeWiseTV and author of the Lifewise Menu Planning System, Faith Hill

In my opinion, Dr. Chance Haugen is one of the most impressive doctors. In a world where money and greed seem to be taking over all decision-making, you find a rare gem such as Dr. Haugen. To understand the weight of what you are learning in this book, you must realize the profoundness of his journey.

Dr. Haugen is a relentless truth seeker for himself, his family and his patients. He lives in a town of approximately 2,000 people. Trust me, I know this because I visited him. He found himself in a health crisis that surpassed the extent of his knowledge through his doctorate and he wanted to know why. In his pursuit of finding true health and the underlying causes of his symptoms, he found Health Centers of the Future. At the time I was a traveling coach for this organization and it led me to traveling to Ortonville to train him and his team on the integration of what he is going to share with you. In my experience I had never seen a doctor with more drive and ambition to get the truth out to the masses. His only (seeming) challenge was that his town did not have the masses. That did not stop him. Dr. Haugen soon began traveling to every nearby town to share the life-changing message that you are so fortunate to find in your hands today.

You will find this book massively refreshing as he so vulnerably and boldly puts the details (including his own lab work) of his case for you to see. You will find him incredibly relatable and down to earth. He was raised a farm boy, so you will have scientific evidence laced with farming analogies to help you understand this complex message. His unique perspective is sure to teach you in a fun and comprehensive way. Dr. Haugen made sure to incorporate all learning styles in this work, as he is dedicated to everyone understanding and believing this information. He has loaded this book with reference studies from Harvard and other respected establishments, all sources referenced for the scientifically inclined. He has also catered to all of you visual learners as well by placing video tutorial links throughout the entire book. Dr. Haugen wants every learning style to grasp this important message.

I call my viewer audience, Total Wellbeings™, because that is what they are! They are fascinated with wellness in all aspects of health from mind, body and relationships. This book is a must have for anyone discovering their Total Wellbeing™. Dr. Haugen thoroughly covers all topics of current ailments that most Americans are facing. Perhaps my favorite two chapters are 18 and 19. I am a firm believer that if you or someone you know is resonating with this book; you are feeling all kinds of emotions at once. There is hope. Dr. Haugen's story along with the other testimonies of total recovery found in chapter 18 will keep you going. As a matter of fact, I recommend starting there if you are facing a chronic health concern right now. After you read chapter 18, then go straight to 19, where Dr. Haugen lays out the simple steps to take action. Once you take action and know help is on the way, go back and read through the rest of this life-changing information to find out why and how your body is in the state of "dis-ease" you find it in. The information you are about to receive has the potential to change your life forever. The deciding factor is you. Read. Take action. Live the life you dream.

Introduction

This book contains the information I used to get my health and my life back. I have been very blessed to have access to some of the best alternative health care doctors in the country. I learned quickly that if you want to learn how to do something, in my case that was getting well, then go find the person who does it best. Don't waste time re-inventing the wheel and trying to figure everything out by yourself. You only have so much time on this earth. I want to share all of the knowledge I have accumulated over the years, but first I want you to know a few things about this book.

First, I've tried to make it very interactive so you can go deeper into the content. There will be access to several deeper level trainings, be sure to take advantage of them.

Second, this book is to help you find out what may be driving inflammation and disease in your body. You don't know what is going on, but you know you're not well. This book will give you ideas as to why that might be.

Third, it is for implementers. You will see that there are lots of ways to start improving your health today. If you're the type who's looking for some magic pill or potion, this isn't the book for you. I'm not here to suggest some gimmick that will make you instantly better.

Fourth, this book isn't intended to agree with everything you think you know. Some things you may never have heard before or some things might seem odd to you. This is not mainstream medical advice and it may conflict with some knowledge you think you know. It's why we call it alternative medicine. Things obviously are not working with what you are doing right now so keep an open mind and I'll think you'll be surprised by the results you get.

Fifth, this book is designed to help you start a conversation, a conversation that will help you start to look at your health deeper and realize how the world around you is affecting you.

Sixth, I don't like books that ramble and so I try to get straight to the point in this book so I can give you a good overview of as many things as possible. I want it to read easily and quickly. If you want to go deeper then utilize the free video trainings available to you.

Seventh, this is a book that is packed with content and lots of ideas. It's a WHAT book, not a step-by-step HOW TO book. My intention and the purpose of this book are to show you the biggest things in your life that are driving inflammation and disease. I want you to understand some of the processes that happen in your body that allow diseases to develop. We have a system available that includes everything you need to eliminate these inflammation and disease drivers from your life.

I'll be the first to admit, I want to help you overcome the health challenges that are costing you money, destroying your relationships, and taking away your precious time. You'll notice there are opportunities throughout this book to register and watch videos and, YES, I do have some great products I'd like to sell to you because they work and you'll have a better life with them.

Table of Contents

Chapter 1-My Story

When I was about 22 years old I started to have all of these odd, unusual symptoms. It started with what seemed like my pulse beating out of my neck. I then started to develop irritable bowel type symptoms. Groin pain came next and night sweats followed. Fatigue was getting worse and I just didn't really want to get up in the morning and go to class. I knew I needed to see a doctor when the groin pain got worse and I started to worry about testicular cancer. I decided I better go and get checked.

I went in. The doctor told me that I had an inflamed prostate. He put me on antibiotics for two months. After those two months went by the symptoms didn't get any better. In fact, they got a little bit worse. He didn't really know what was going on. He decided to send me to a specialist. He sent me to a urologist first. He did an ultrasound, checking out different areas, making sure everything was okay. That came back fine. He then referred me on to someone else. They ordered a CT scan. The CT scan came back fine. Nothing was wrong on there. I started to slowly question the doctors and whether or not they knew what they were doing.

I was living away from home at the time and I wanted to go back to a clinic that knew me and my history so I scheduled a visit back home with a doctor. He actually recommended a colonoscopy. When he looked at the colonoscopy, he said, "Everything looks fine in the colon, except I see something that doesn't have a medical explanation. I see what appear to be little bugs or parasites. There's nothing we can do for it and I doubt it is causing your problems. I see it from time to time." I thought this doc was nuts and decided to move on. I ended up back at the original doctor, wanting to know where I could go next or what I should do. He said, "Let's do a culture."
I said, "Fine." At this point, I just wanted some answers.
He said, "If something is wrong, we'll call you. If nothing is wrong, you'll just get a letter in the mail."
A couple weeks later I got a letter in the mail and the letter said, "Your vaginal pap smear was normal." Now, that might be funny right now but at

the time you can imagine just how upset I was. That was my last straw with the medical system, I was completely fed up.

I decided to go to a chiropractor. Now, when I went to the chiropractor, he said, "Well, let's take an X-ray of your spine."
I said, "There's nothing wrong with my spine, my back doesn't hurt, why are we going to look at my spine? My back doesn't hurt."
He said, "Let's just take a look." We took a look. I found out I had a curvature in my thoracic and lumbar spine. I had no idea it was there. He said. "Some of these symptoms are probably coming from nerve pressure because of the curvature."
I said, "All right." I was desperate by this time and went through a care plan. Three or four weeks later, a lot of my symptoms got way better. My digestion improved. The groin pain was gone. All of those things left; I felt a lot better.

What continued on after that was my fatigue. I couldn't lose weight. I actually started to gain more and more and more weight. I got to 235 pounds at my heaviest which I had never seen before. I was at 200 before all of the issues started. It didn't matter how little I ate, how much I exercised, I couldn't seem to lose any pounds and this was very, very frustrating for me. I just couldn't figure it out. I tried all kinds of things to get better. I'd take a supplement and see if it would help, if it didn't I would move on and try the next one. I'd diet for a period of time. I would eat very few calories, cut way back on my fat intake and still no results. I exercised for months with no results. I would get a little bit better with some of the strategies I tried, but never truly got well.

This went on for three or four years. I started to develop new health issues which included a fungus on my feet. It looked like athlete's foot and I just couldn't get rid of it. I ended up having it for 3 straight years, with it never leaving. It didn't matter what cream or powder I put on it. At noon, when I would be adjusting people, I would actually have to lay down for a half hour or an hour each and every day just to make it through my days of adjusting people. I couldn't take it. That's how bad the fatigue was. Finally, my brother said in all of his wisdom, "Why don't you pray about it?" I started to pray and asked for answers.

The answers started to come. A doctor advertised an event on Facebook and I decided I needed to go. I had never even heard of this doctor or event before, but I liked what I heard in the ad so I went. Everything that he said absolutely made sense for once. I made up mind at that time. I didn't care how much it cost. I didn't care what I had to do. I was going to get well. I made that choice. What I'm going to share with you here in this book is everything that I've learned throughout the years. I've trained and learned from some of the best alternative doctors in the country. Inflammation is at the core root of disease and when you find what is causing the inflammation it will begin to leave your body. When inflammation leaves your body it can finally do what it was designed to do, get well.

I started my journey with different types of strategic fasting because I knew I had to fix my digestion first if I wanted to get well. My digestive issues started to get better with the fasts. I also noticed that my feet were starting to heal and that the fungus was leaving. I took a meta-oxy inflammation test and it came back at the highest level possible for inflammation. I knew I had work to do. I cut out all grains and sugar from my diet to stop the inflammation in its tracks. My energy was slowly starting to come back. I started to look at other areas of my life where I could reduce toxins. I had a heavy metal urine challenged test performed and it showed high amounts of mercury and lead. I had my amalgams removed by an IAOMT dentist and started to do oral chelation. Three months into chelation I passed a huge amount of parasites. Turns out the doctor who did my colonoscopy was right. I immediately started to lose more weight, my clarity came back and my irritability started to decrease. I kept using different fasts and burst training to help me burn toxic fat. I was able to start exercising again without feeling tired for days. I was getting my life back. My wife could see the difference and started to find ways to cook healthier and find clean food. We started to remove chemicals in our house including cleaning products and personal care products. We continue to learn and find new ways to clean up our life.
I'm going to show you through this book the biggest culprits that are affecting your health and how you can find them in your own life. What you choose to do with the information is up to you, but I know that if you start implementing what we teach you can get the same results.

Chapter 2-Inflammation

We had a go cart when I was a kid and my neighbor also had a go cart. We lived out in the country and had a lot of room to roam. We would play cops and robbers with the go carts and chase each other. We would drive all over the farm and have a blast. One day we came around a big evergreen tree and we couldn't see each other and we hit head on. His go cart jumped up on top of mine and smashed into my ankle. I immediately knew something was wrong. My ankle swelled up instantly and I couldn't put any weight on it. Luckily I didn't break anything and just had to be on crutches for a week. I recovered after a few weeks and I was back to normal. What if the inflammation hadn't gone down, what if the inflammation became chronic? Can you imagine? It would have interrupted my life and caused a lot of problems. This is actually happening to a lot of us, but it is happening at the cellular level in our bodies.

To understand inflammation I think we need to get the definition of inflammation first. Now when I say inflammation most of you may automatically think of the redness or swelling around a cut or a sprained ankle like in my go cart accident, the swelling, bruising, and inability for the joint to move. Or maybe it's the inflammation associated with joint pain and arthritis. These are all inflammatory processes, but I also want to look at something known as chronic inflammation, not just acute.

This definition is from the Miller-Keane Encyclopedia and Dictionary of Medicine, Nursing and Allied Health. Here's what they say, "Inflammation is a localized protective response elicited by injury or destruction of tissues, which serves to destroy, dilute, or wall off both the injurious agent and the injured tissue. Inflammatory response can be provoked by physical, chemical and biological agents, including mechanical trauma, exposure to excessive amounts of sunlight, x-rays and radioactive materials, corrosive chemicals, extremes of heat and cold, or by infectious agents such as bacteria, viruses, and other pathogenic microorganisms. Although these infectious agents can produce inflammation, infection and inflammation are not synonymous. The classic gns of inflammation are heat, redness, swelling, pain and loss of function. These are manifestations of physiological changes that occur during the inflammatory process. The three major components of this process are changes in the caliber of the blood vessels and the rate of blood flow through them, increased capillary permeability and leukocytic exudation."

Now it goes on after this in a lot more detail, things that I don't think we need to cover because only a biochemist will understand half of the language. I think we really get kind of the overall picture of inflammation here. There are some things I want to go back and talk about, so if you noticed in that first line it talks about it serves to destroy both whatever is causing the inflammation and the injured tissue. Not only is the body trying to get rid of whatever's making it sick, it's also destroying tissue in your body. Now imagine if this is chronic inflammation. That means that your body is trying to destroy its own tissue all the time. This is a really big deal. This is how autoimmune disease can stem from chronic inflammation. Autoimmune disease basically means that your body continually attacks itself. A great way to picture this is from a movie scene in *Liar Liar* where Jim Carrey beats the crap out of himself in the bathroom. Picture that every time you think of autoimmune disease, your body beating itself up. Until you get rid of the inflammation it will continue to do so. There are over 200 identified autoimmune conditions and the list continues to grow. Here is a list of common autoimmune illnesses and illnesses linked to autoimmune problems in the body.

Celiac Disease
Cancer
Crohns
Colitis
IBS
Cushings/Addison's
Hashimotos/Graves
Leaky Gut
Type 1 Diabetes
Eczema
Psoriasis
Endometriosis

Rheumatoid
Lupus
Scleroderma
Autism
Type 2 Diabetes
Weight loss resistance
Brain Fog and Memory Loss
Hair Loss
Food Allergies
Arthritis

It is well-known that decreasing inflammation in the body can help with all of these diseases, that is why for a majority of them doctors use anti-inflammatory medications.

Now let's go back to that inflammation definition and what I want to point out here is that it says it can be provoked by physical, chemical and biological agents. It's not just one thing; there are a lot of things that cause inflammation.

I believe it can also be provoked by emotions. We'll talk about that later in the book. But you can get an overall picture here of what happens when inflammation strikes. It can come from a lot of different angles and it can cause a lot of different things to happen in the body that result in a wide range of symptoms and it really is a start of almost every single disease there is in the body.

Inflammation is both good and bad. Acute inflammation is very good; it's trying to protect the body. If you get a sprained ankle, if you get a cut, the body is going there to try to fix the problem. Chronic inflammation is also trying to fix the problem, but it never does. Chronic inflammation is what we need to work on and we need to find out what's causing it in your life because it's going to be different for each individual. You and I don't have the same mothers, the same upbringing, the same house, the same job, etc. Figuring out what is at the root can be difficult, but figuring out how to remove it can be even more work. I'm going to show you how to simplify everything. You'll be able to see what is driving inflammation in your body.

Do you remember cells from science class? How they have mitochondria, ribosomes, membranes, a nucleus, etc. There's a lot that goes on in a cell and inflammation can make it come to a stop. Your cells have to let nutrients in and they have to expel waste. When your body is inflamed it becomes very difficult for this to happen. You can take a lot of supplements and they may not even get to your cells for your body to use. Just because you are taking a multi-vitamin or high doses of a vitamin doesn't mean that your body is using it. If your body is inflamed it will be difficult for it to use. Your cells will also be backing up with toxins because they can't get out through the inflamed cell membrane. Your liver starts to become burdened because it can't keep up. This can lead to fatty liver disease and even gallbladder problems. Cellular inflammation can even lead to hormone problems that so many women struggle with. Your cells have receptors on the outside of them that hormones bind onto. They then send a signal to the cell telling it to do something. If a cell is too inflamed a hormone may not be able to bind to the receptor leading to hormone dysregulation. Reducing cellular inflammation has to be the main goal or the body will not be able to complete its everyday tasks and this is what leads to disease.

If you want to know more about inflammation and how it affects you, I have made a special video series that you can get for free. I draw out a cell and how inflammation affects it. You'll get a much clearer picture of exactly what goes on. Just go to this link and sign up to view them. http://www.inflammationdetox.com/getfreevideos

Chapter 3-Bucket Theory

I want you to picture an old tub in your upstairs slowly filling with water and it doesn't have an overflow drain. One of your kids turned the water on and you have no idea that they did it. At what point are you going to know that your bathtub is filling with water?

You're not going to know there's a problem until it overflows and now you have water spreading out all over the floors and maybe down the stairs and through the ceiling. The same thing is happening in our bodies. This is known as the bucket theory. If you picture all of us having a bucket; our bodies can handle so much at one time and so many exposures at one time—it's made to handle toxins coming in and toxins going out. What we want is to have more toxins going out than coming in.

So what do you do when there are way more toxins coming in than going out? Maybe you're dealing with emotional trauma, a physical injury like a car accident, mold exposure, lead exposure, some heavy metal exposure. All of these things can start to add up in your body, and eventually you can't keep up and your bucket overflows. That's when you get all of these symptoms. Now, if you don't go in and start to clean up and empty that bucket you continuously get that overflow of water or symptoms when we look at it from the perspective of your body. You have to start to clean out that bucket or it's going to continue to overflow.

This is where modern medicine, and even alternative medicine can falter. You can throw the medications, or all the vitamins that you want at those symptoms but until you remove the source of the problem, the bucket is going to continue to overflow. You can cover it up with band aids; you can try to bail the water, but you are never going to catch up with it until you get rid of that source.

A lot of times people will go to an alternative doctor and find out that they are deficient in a certain vitamin or mineral. They may have had a machine, blood, or muscle testing done to determine this. It is great to find out that you are deficient in something and then replenish it, but if you never find out why you were deficient in the first place it is more than likely going to keep re-occurring. One of the biggest issues that I hear people tell me is that they get parasites quite often and have to get rid of them. Well why do they keep re-occurring? Why can't your body get rid of them on its own? More than likely there is something deeper going on that you are missing. There is something in your life that is keeping you from truly being healthy.

Now, in no way are you ever going to stop all the toxins in your life. It's impossible, but you want to drastically reduce them as much as you can and you want to get rid of the main culprits, the ones that you know are there. Turn the faucet down to just a drip. If you can do that your body's going to be able to handle those stressors and those toxins a lot easier. Whether it's physical, chemical, or emotional, all three of them, once again, can cause issues or cause your bucket to overflow.

Throughout the rest of the book I'm going to show you the main culprits filling the bucket and I'm also going to show you how inflammation affects some of the major health issues this country faces. I'll also explain some of the processes as to how inflammation affects the body.

Do you think your bucket is overflowing? Go to this link and watch the videos. I draw the bucket theory and explain it in much greater detail.
http://www.inflammationdetox.com/getfreevideos

Chapter 4-Methylation and Epigenetics

"I probably got that from grandpa or it just runs in the family." We have all said this phrase at least once in our life. When we are talking about diseases and inheriting them from our family members we now know that this is only partially true. Our DNA is not our destiny. We once thought that our DNA made the decisions in our body and that we were stuck with what happened once a gene was turned on or off. Bruce Lipton, a stem cell biologist and author of The Biology of Belief, says it best, "Just like a single cell, the character of our lives is determined not by our genes but by our responses to the environmental signals that propel life."

Epigenetics has shed a whole new light on how our genes actually work. We can change how our genes express themselves through epigenetics. We now know what changes how those genes are expressed. Stressors in our life end up changing our genes. This means that what you eat, the chemicals you ingest, the amount of sleep you get, and how you control your emotions all affect your genes. Let's look at BPA for example. BPA is a chemical found in some plastics and has been banned in baby bottles and it's hard to find a water container now that doesn't say BPA free on it. This is for a good reason. We know that when you ingest BPA it goes to the cell and turns on a fat gene. If nothing is done to turn the fat gene off then then any offspring are also going to have that gene turned on. This is how you can say that you did indeed get it from a family member, but we also know that you have the power to turn that gene off again by following the right steps. You can change your genes through something called methylation. Methylation is a part of many processes in the body.

- It is a vital part of epigenetics(turning genes on and off)
- It protects and stabilizes DNA
- It helps with stress adaptation by activating and deactivating stress hormones
- It affects your mood because it activates serotonin, melatonin, and dopamine
- Energy production
- Detoxification

- Gowth and healing
- Autonomic nervous system,
- Immune system
- It is involved in every aspect of the disease process.

Pretty important processes as you can see. When you become methyl depleted it can lead to many unexplainable conditions such as

- Chronic Fatigue
- Sleep Disorders
- Inability to adapt to stress
- Toxic Encephalitis
- Genetic Disorders
- Hormone Dysregulation
- Cancer
- Weight Loss Resistance

We have to have methyl groups to function properly. Everything that we talk about later in the book will deplete your body of methyl groups—diet, malabsorption, toxins, stress, and hormone dysregulation.

Survival is always the body's most instinctive and immediate need. During a stressor the body will use methyl groups to activate stress hormones adrenaline and cortisol. Once the body has handled the stress it will deactivate adrenaline and cortisol. Then it will maintain everyday bodily function. If it has enough methyl groups it will help the body repair and heal(even DNA). If there are still enough methyl groups it will store it for energy. This is a list of priorities that the body has so if you don't have enough methyl groups many of these processes may not be happening in your body. If you have a chronic stress in your life that is depleting methyl groups this is where disease can start. The body is so focused on that immediate stressor that other bodily functions might not be happening like DNA protection. This is how cancer and premature aging can start. Or maybe there are not enough methyl groups to remove toxic estrogen metabolites and this leads to cancer. There are so many diseases that can happen because of methyl depletion. For instance people with the CYP2D629B+ gene have a three times likelihood of developing dementia along with Parkinsons disease. MNSOD/NQ01 – these two genes give you a four fold increase in Parkinsons disease. However, the studies show that the genes alone do not cause Parkinsons disease. It is the environmental triggers that initiate the illness.

If you want to learn more about methylation and its role in the body visit http://www.inflammationdetox.com/getfreevideos

Chapter 5-The Gut-Where It All Starts

When my problems first started I had never had digestive issues in my life and it was odd to me that it came out of nowhere. The more I learned about the gut the more I knew I had to fix it or I would never get well. The antibiotics that I took for 2 months, that were supposed to help my inflamed prostate, destroyed all of my gut bacteria. Gut bacteria actually help regulate hormones for hunger and an unbalance can lead to weight gain. This is why I started to gain weight out of nowhere. Once I started to correct the bacteria in my stomach it made everything else a lot easier.

Do you ever feel lethargic after you eat a meal? Feel bloated, have low energy, just can't seem to concentrate? Do you regularly like you should just take a nap? This is how strong our gut and our brain are connected. You have more neurons in your gut than you do in your spinal cord or your peripheral nervous system. You literally feel what is going on in your gut. The gut actually does some of its own work without the brains help. In fact your vagus nerve, the primary nerve to your gut, sends about 90% of its information from the gut to the brain, not the other way around. If your gut is inflamed your brain is inflamed. This can lead to depression, anxiety, and life altering energy levels that keep us stuck in a rut. If you do not fix gut issues it is extremely hard if not impossible to get well. How can we start to work on this? Your gut will not heal itself overnight. There are over 100 trillion organisms living in your gut. You have more bacteria in your gut than you do cells in our body. Who is controlling who? We have 25,000 genes; they have 3.3 million. These bacteria make up 70-80% of our immune system.

Balancing and replenishing these good bacteria can help calm the inflammation in our gut. Fermented foods, which mean that the food has living bacteria on/in it can help us start to get some of these good guys back in our guts. Probiotic supplements are ok, but they don't come close to being as beneficial as fermented foods.
The gut is the gateway to the body. Leaky gut is an alternative medicine term. Leaky gut is when your gut allows things like proteins, toxins,

bacteria, etc. to leak across the lining of your intestines and into your bloodstream. This can trigger an autoimmune response in your body. This can manifest as bloating, excessive gas and cramps, weight gain, fatigue, food sensitivities, joint pain, skin rashes, and autoimmunity.

To show you how leaky gut can affect your health I'd like to tell you about my experiences with it. Early on when my body was healing if I ate grains for a day or two straight my body would start to react and become inflamed. Grains contain proteins that can leak across the gut; the most famous protein is gluten, but there are others. My digestion would be terrible, my wrists and forearms would start to ache, my lower back would get sore, athletes foot would start to reappear on my feet, and my energy would tank.The only way I could break that was to change my food and start to take things that would allow my gut lining to heal. Most people don't even realize how their gut is affecting them until they make some of these changes, and then they see how life altering it can be.

So how can you start to see changes in your gut? You have to give it time and you have to give it the right food. Fasting is one of the most important tools in allowing the gut to regenerate. Intermittent fasting is one of my favorites. This allows the body time to heal without having to digest food. I also have patients fast with fermented foods like cultured whey; Socrates called it healing water. This allows the body to take a break from digesting and it also gives the body beneficial bacteria that can start rebuilding in the gut. Fasting with bone broth is another great tool we use that allows the gut to start regenerating.

After you have worked on the gut you can start to move on to other areas that need attention. You will see big changes just with gut work.

If you are having digestive issues and want to learn more follow the link below.
http://www.inflammationdetox.com/getfreevideos

Chapter 6-Bad Fats

Whenever I needed to lose a little weight when I was young I just cut way back on my calories, stayed with low fat foods and spent a few extra minutes on the treadmill. It seemed to work and I could drop 5-10 pounds in no time. When I got sick that all changed. Cutting the calories, fat and exercising more did nothing. It was so frustrating. I was following the advice that we were all given at one point in time. It turns out that this is not great advice and that the scientific literature says to do something completely different.

I grew up on a farm and I learned how to change oil in a lot of different machinery. The oil kept everything well lubricated and the engine running smooth. If you used the wrong oil or didn't change it regularly it was going to cause a lot of problems. The same can be said about the oil or fat that you are putting in your body and more than likely you are in need of an oil change.

Many oils/fats can cause our engines to dysfunction and eventually even cause death. It is vital we are putting the right oil into our body and change that oil if we are using the wrong ones right now.

This can also be a challenge for some people because they do not want to change how they eat. If you don't change you don't get well, it is that simple. Change can be a lot easier than you think. The best thing you can do is think about your favorite foods and find replacements for them. First, though we have to define what is good and what is bad. Let's start with the bad and what you must cut out. The first thing that we're going to look is bad fats. Why? Because you can implement this immediately and it doesn't take a lot of work or skill. Basically what we've been told, by our government and health experts is that we need to eat less because we're gluttons; we need to exercise more to lose weight because we're too lazy; we need to avoid fats and eat more whole grains. It's common sense.

That's what we're told all the time. Eat less; exercise more. Think about the housewives in the 1950s. Do you think those 1950s housewives were out running triathlons and marathons, and getting in their three mile runs every single day? I don't think so. Did we have the huge weight problem, hormone issues, and cancer rates skyrocketing? Obesity rates have risen over 20% since 1950.

Growing up everyone told us to stay away from fat. We were told that fats were giving us heart disease, cancer, and strokes. The truth is fats have gotten a really, really bad rap. Fat does not make you fat. It's the inability to burn fat that makes you fat and sick.

In fact, good fats are actually going to help you burn fat and make you healthier. What we've been told is that an increase in dietary fat increases our LDL, our cholesterol, and our chance for cardiovascular disease. The truth is that increased sugar intake, and an increase in bad fats drives inflammation in our arteries and drives heart disease.

This is an area that was a huge concern for me, and something that I really had to look into. My grandpa died of a heart attack when I was five years old; my other grandfather had many strokes and ultimately died from them. My uncles have had heart attacks and strokes. My grandmother has had a heart attack. Heart disease is really prevalent in my family so this is something that is very important to me. I know it's of huge importance to a lot of Americans just because heart disease is still our number one killer.

The reason we're not seeing a change is because we're looking at this picture wrong, like fat is still an enemy; it's not. Inflammation is the enemy here so we have to decrease inflammation in the body.

There's a difference between good fat, and bad fat. We want to eliminate bad fats, and we want to increase good fats. The reason we want to eliminate bad fats is because they drive inflammation and oxidative stress. When I say oxidation, think of something like rust. That's what bad fats will do; they'll drive that inflammation and build up plaque/rust in your arteries. This oxidation in your arteries will then lead to heart disease and other inflammatory problems.

Man-made fats are usually the culprit when it comes to bad fats—bad fats, such as hydrogenated vegetable oils, partially hydrogenated oils, trans-fats, and rancid vegetable oils. Oils that have been processed like canola oil, are no longer good. Margarine is a bad man-made processed fat.

Drop the bad fats and increase the good like saturated fat. I know it goes against everything you've been told. The article in the June 2014 issue of *Time Magazine*, "Eat Butter. Scientists Labeled Fat the Enemy, Why They Were Wrong." has been a huge revelation and we're starting to realize that butter isn't the enemy, saturated fat isn't the enemy.

If you go all the way back to 1961, the cover of *Time Magazine* had Ancel Keys on it. He claimed that, "Saturated fats and high fat diets clogged arteries and caused heart disease." The Time cover from March of 1984 says, "Cholesterol, and Now the Bad News." We were told to eat low fat diets for 50 years and it has caused diseases in this country to skyrocket.

There are so many good fats that you can start using right away—coconut oil, butter, grapeseed oil, MCT oil, etc. Here's a tip for you when you use these oils: When you cook you have to be careful not to turn these fats rancid. Some fats don't do very well with heat and some do great at high heat. When you are cooking with heat make sure you are using stable oil.

Here are some studies that have been done that show the importance of fat.

A 2009 study from Harvard School of Public Health showed the more vegetable oils, the women in the study ate, the worse their atherosclerosis became. The irony of the study was the more saturated fat they ate the less their atherosclerosis progressed. The highest levels of saturated fat, actually even started to reverse some of those conditions over time.[10] Numerous studies show bad fats cause inflammation in the cell membrane which can lead to type 2 diabetes.

The Nurse's Health Study showed a substantial reduction of type 2 diabetes when good fats were added, and trans-fats were reduced. Eighty-four thousand nurses took part in the study. The total saturated fat intakes were not associated with an increased risk of diabetes, only the trans-fat.[2] The Harvard showed a diet high in saturated fats from meats and dairy improved diabetes three-fold.[1]

The University of Pittsburgh study indicated that frequent users of partially hydrated vegetable oils had higher insulin levels.[3] Bad fats cause inflammation of the cell, blunting hormone receptors and driving autoimmune disease because of the inflammation.[4] It heightens the immune response, so studies show a diet high in vegetable oils which turn rancid during processing decreased thyroid function by causing inflammation.[5]

The Volek Study and other show that diets high in saturated fat and low in carbs improved weight loss by improving thyroid function. The diet and the study had fifty percent of calories from good fat, low in carbs, and moderate amounts of protein.[4] A study looking at tolerance to cold compared diets high in protein, carbs, and fat, it was only the diet high in saturated fat, due to its effect on the thyroid that improved tolerance to cold.[6]

To learn more about good fats and bad fats follow this link to a free video series. http://www.inflammationdetox.com/getfreevideos

Chapter 7-Sugar

Mountain Dew. I used to love it, if I could have drunk one thing it would have been Mountain Dew. I stopped drinking it when I got sick because I really tried to cut sugar out of my diet and when I came back to it I couldn't believe how sweet it tasted, I didn't even like it anymore. It is amazing how your taste buds can change once you get away from sugar. One of the treats that we have in the house now is 60% cacao chocolate chips. If you would have had me try one before I quit sugar I would have told you that they tasted a little blah, but now I think they taste great! Making these changes won't be as hard as you think; finding the right replacements will help you overcome your addiction.

Your body uses two things for energy. It can either burn sugar or it can burn fat. Most of America is stuck in sugar burning mode. Their body doesn't have the ability to go back and forth between burning sugar and burning fat. When your body cannot burn fat because of inflamed hormone receptors it will give you cravings to eat sugar. It will utilize this as its energy source. I'd like you to understand why your body is stuck using only sugar and how you can change that and become a fat burning machine.

When a type 2 diabetic has problems with blood sugar it is because their cell is too inflamed to hear the hormone insulin. Insulin is responsible for opening a gate so glucose is able to go into the cell, which keeps your blood sugar normal. Well when a cell starts to become inflamed or damaged, it now has fewer places for insulin to bind onto that cell, less gates open for glucose to get into the cell so your blood sugar starts to rise, you start to become hormone resistant to insulin.

This is very similar to what happens with the hormone leptin. Leptin is the hormone that controls food cravings and fat burning in your body. When scientists discovered this they thought that they were going to be able to make a lot of money, they were going to be able to just give people leptin and they were going to burn a lot of fat and lose weight.

What they found is that people who are overweight already have plenty of leptin, in fact, they have too much. The fact is that people weren't able to hear the leptin in their body because their cells were so blunted and so inflamed, so their body's producing leptin telling them to stop eating, telling them to burn fat, but the cells can't hear it so nothing is happening, and they become hormone resistant.

A lot of illnesses develop in a very similar in this way. Many thyroid problems are a result of the inability to hear your thyroid hormone; diabetes, the inability of the cell to hear insulin. Obesity has a lot to do with the inability to hear leptin. These hormone resistance problems are due to inflammation of the cell.

Getting sugar out of your diet can help with a lot of hormone related problems and will dramatically decrease inflammation in your body.

To learn more about how sugar can blunt hormone receptors you can go here and watch these free videos.
http://www.inflammationdetox.com/getfreevideos

Chapter 8-Grains

How many of you remember the old Food Pyramid? We were all told that we should be eating whole grains the most out of any food group. I know growing up that became a staple of our diet. We would have grains at every single meal. What if I told you that the food pyramid could basically be flipped upside down and you and your family would be a lot healthier? Your kids would have better concentration in school because they wouldn't have a sugar crash half way through the morning because of all the grains they eat at breakfast. Now they've changed the food pyramid into something called My Plate. They don't even have a fat category anymore and I just showed you how important those are earlier. My Plate is no better than the Food Pyramid.

Now a lot of you look at me like whole grains? Really? How can you compare that to sugar? In fact, I think that whole grains are actually worse than sugar because the truth is that two slices of whole wheat toast increase your blood sugar more than five to six teaspoons of pure sugar. That's the same as drinking a whole can of soda. When you get up in the morning and you eat those two pieces of toast you immediately are spiking your blood sugar and it stays sustained longer than it would if you ate pure sugar .

This is why grains have to be cut out if you want to get well. Now I'm not saying all grains are terrible. I'm just saying in order to decrease inflammation in your body they have to be cut out for the time being because they turn to sugar so easily in your body.

Grains have been hybridized and crossbred to be the addictive super sugar that they are. Norman Borlaug wanted to solve world hunger, and he had a great idea, won the Nobel Prize for it, but what we never did was test what was going to happen when we made this new wheat. Now we're starting to see the consequences, world obesity. We have new hybrids now and they're higher in sugar and they're more addictive. What happens if you try to go off of grains for a while? You get withdrawal symptoms and cravings. It's very similar to a drug. It won't take too long to break the habit, four or five days and the cravings really slow down and stop.

The new gluten in wheat has gone through many structural changes due to hybridizations and we've created fourteen new gluten proteins that weren't in either parent wheat. There are now thousands of new strains without any safety testing. However, it's not just gluten in the wheat, there are other denatured proteins in wheat as well, and there are also phytates and lectins which are toxic anti-nutrients in all grains and they increase inflammation. To get well we need to take grains out for the time being. Once you've reached your health goals, there are healthy grains that you can add back to your diet, but not in the amount that you are consuming them right now.

You know it's funny, one of the most overlooked things I see when someone comes in from another doctor and they say they've been working on getting to the source of their problem is that they've never looked at their diet. They've been on all these supplements and all these medications, and they've tried so many different things, but no one has shown them how to change their diet. If you don't make these dietary changes it's going to be almost impossible for you to get well.

If you want to learn more about how to cut grains out of your diet and why you need to, go here and watch this free video series.
http://www.inflammationdetox.com/getfreevideos

Chapter 9-Toxins

When most people think of toxins or they think of a toxic source they may think of some sort of really bad chemical spill or a radioactive material. One of the most well-known toxic sources that people really know and relate to is smoking. Everyone knows how bad smoking is for you. It can cause lung cancer, heart disease, and many other illnesses. How do all of those diseases start? They start with inflammation from the chemicals in the cigarette. I want everyone to see that all of these diseases start with inflammation in the body and if you remove the chemical it stops the inflammatory process. I'm going to cover the biggest offenders in this section and by no means will I cover all of them. These will also be some of the easiest changes you can make.

We all agree that smoking exposes us to toxins; what else exposes us to toxins? Let's look at this a little bit. Merriam Webster defines toxic as: "containing or being poisonous material, especially when capable of causing death or serious debilitation or it may be extremely harsh, malicious or harmful exhibiting symptoms, infection or toxicosis." I'm going to go through and show you what I believe are the toxins affecting most Americans right now.

Every toxic element is going to have an upper limit of normal or what's safe to consume. Whether we're talking about a heavy metal like lead or mercury or maybe fluoride, chlorine, or bromine; whether we're talking about things like BPA or chemicals in plastics, all of these things are said to be safe in certain amounts, but once they reach a certain limit they become toxic. It becomes too much for a body to handle. A lot of these elements we're unable to process or get rid of, and that's the hard part. When these exposures become chronic at what point do they start causing harm?

Plastics can be toxic, especially those containing BPA, which the FDA banned from baby bottles; but plastics have a huge effect on our health and on our hormones especially. In a recent study published in Plus One Journal[7], German researchers found that there were nearly twenty-five thousand chemicals lurking in a single bottle of water. They showed that amounts as little as .01 ounce prohibited estrogenic activity by 60% and androgenic activity by 90%. This means that their hormones were dramatically changed. When hormones change in the body it can lead to cancers and many other dangerous diseases.

Fluoride's a controversial subject in this country. On the CDC's website they warn if you get too much fluoride exposure it can lead to bone loss and it can also even lead to dental fluorosis. Now at what limit does that start to happen in the body? Do you want to take a chance of continually being exposed to fluoride throughout the course of your life and do you think it's worth it? Those are questions that you have to ask yourself. If you ever do have questions concerning a substance and wonder if there are studies about it, I encourage you to visit websites like PubMed.gov. For Example, you could type in "fluoride toxicity" and look at all of the studies available on that subject; very useful tool.

Fluoride is also in a group called halogens. If you remember that scientific table from science class, fluoride, bromine and chlorine all fall into that group. Well they all act very similarly because of their make-up. Fluoride and halogens have an affinity for the thyroid because iodine is also a halogen. We all know that we need iodine for our thyroid to work. Well if you have low levels of iodine or you're iodine deficient, those levels of fluoride, chlorine, or bromine could have an effect on your thyroid. This is something you need to look at and decide for yourself if these chemicals are something that you want to put into your body.

You'll notice if you turn over your toothpaste tube there is a warning on the back, if swallowed contact a poison control center. That small amount of toothpaste is enough to warrant a call to a poison control center.

Chlorine was used in WWI as a choking or pulmonary agent in chemical weapons. We now put chlorine in all of our drinking water and it's in our pools. We know that chlorine has toxic effects and is very toxic to us in high concentrations. What about low concentrations over a long period of time, chronic exposure? Once again, these are questions you have to ask yourself and decide if it's worth the exposure.

The most toxic appliance in a persons home is probably their dishwasher. Most people have never considered this and for good reason. Now what makes your dishwasher so toxic? Well if you live in the city you have chlorine and fluoride going in the dishwasher. You have the detergent with all the chemicals in there. What happens when you open that dishwasher up? Boom! A cloud of toxic gas right? It fills the whole house and everyone gets to enjoy that chemical fume. The fastest way to your bloodstream is through your lungs. Those chemicals will start to affect bodily processes immediately.

If your dishwasher is releasing this toxic gas, then that means there is one more area of your home where you are breathing this gas in as well. Nice long hot showers.

Bromine is another one that's in that class of halogens. Bromine is normally used as a flame retardant. It's found on your furniture and bed; it's replaced iodine in bread. Bromine is also in a lot of soft drinks. It's another one of those exposures that you can eliminate easily yourself. It's also used in pools and hot tubs. It is unnecessary and you can now find non-toxic agents for your pool and hot tub. Again, you have to ask yourself, are these exposures worth it or do I want to start eliminating these from my life and start to maybe clean some of this stuff up?

Household cleaners. This should be a given—if you're using household cleaners that aren't clean, please start to replace them, start to get green ones. I'll tell you, they work great, and do just as good of a job. Toxic chemicals like formaldehyde, ethylbenzene, petroleum distillate, petroleum chemicals, chlorine, benzine are very common in cleaners—I'm not going to go into how these all affect you, but you can just see how many toxins are in a lot of these cleaners, and we have to start getting them out.

We already discussed how dishwashing detergents can become gas and enter your bloodstream. The same thing can happen with oven cleaners. Laundry detergent chemicals can end up on your skin through direct contact with your clothes. You can also breathe in the chemicals all day that end up on your clothes after they've been washed.

Air fresheners can be extremely toxic. Yeah, they make your house smell better but, there are plenty of products out there that freshen your air and aren't going to release a ton of chemical toxins into the air.

Antibacterial cleaners and soaps may contain triclosan. In my home state of Minnesota they've actually banned this in soap because they know how toxic it is.

I can remember when my wife and I got to buy new furniture for our house for the very first time in our lives. We had the couch picked out and went up to purchase the product. As we went through the process the lady who sold us the couch asked us if we wanted to have a stain resistant spray put on it. I kindly said no because I didn't think we would have any issues with spilling things on it and she said that if we planned on having kids that I might want to reconsider. I thought about it for a minute and asked her what was in the spray. She went on to say how it was safe and they used it all the time. I debated in my own head and finally decided not to have it done. When I got home I looked up the spray and found that it was anything but free from toxic chemicals.

A lot of parents have their furniture sprayed so their kids don't spill things all over them and ruin them. I know firsthand the destruction that can happen with kids, but be aware of what you're putting on there and what you're going to be having your skin touching, what your kids are going to be licking, biting, and chewing. How will those chemicals affect your child's body?

Mattresses can be a big offender as well. Make sure they're not being sprayed with a bunch of flame retardants, because you're spending a third of your day on them and if they're off-gassing you're going to be breathing it in. There are many safe mattresses that are made out things like wool, kevlar, and many others.

Pesticides. There are numerous studies that link pesticide use to health problems, but I like this one because I grew up on a farm and it shows that you don't have to be the user of the pesticide to be affected by it. Women married to men who use pesticides have almost a two fold increase in thyroid disease.[8]

Food and chemical additives. You have to start to be aware of your food and food that drives inflammation. So we talked about bad fats, sugars, grains, and how they drive inflammation. But there's also a lot of food out there that is sprayed with pesticides, sweetened with unhealthy artificial sweeteners like aspartame, or laced with excitotoxins like MSG. I'm not saying you have to eat organic for everything, but some foods are a lot worse than others.

Makeup. A woman starts her morning with an average of 515 different chemicals. It is no wonder women are struggling with an unprecedented number of hormone health issues. Here's one of the first places you should start looking, your natural care products.
According to the Safe Cosmetics Campaign, you should avoid the following chemicals in cosmetics whenever possible:

Butyl acetate
Butylated hydroxytoluene
Coal tar
Cocamide DEA/lauramide DEA
Diazolidinyl urea
Ethyl acetate
Formaldehyde
Parabens (methyl, ethyl, propyl and butyl)
Petrolatum
Phthalates
Propylene glycol
Sodium laureth/sodium laurel sulfate Talc
Toluene
Triethanolamine

I tried to list the easiest toxins in your life that you can start removing right now. If you want to learn more about others that might be affecting you then please follow this link to get more answers.
http://www.inflammationdetox.com/getfreevideos

Chapter 10-Heavy Metals

I believe that a heavy metal detox can be one of the most rewarding detoxes, but it can also be one of the most dangerous if done incorrectly. With so many heavy metals how do we know if we are being affected by them or if we have chronic levels in our body? When I was sick I decided to look at heavy metals to see if they might be affecting my health and filling my bucket up quicker. Getting the right test done is very important. We want to look at chronic levels of metals in our body and a blood test would only show an acute exposure.The body holds on to the metals tightly and they begin to bioaccumulate in our organs and tissue. There is no perfect heavy metal test, but I believe a urine challenge test gives you the best look at your chronic levels.

I was shocked when I came back with high levels of lead and high levels of mercury. I didn't understand where the exposure came from so I started to do some research. The number one source for lead exposure is actually from a mother during pregnancy. I tested my mom to see if this might be the source of my exposure. I was shocked by what I found. Her lead levels were off the chart and her mercury levels were also high. I believe most of my exposure actually came from her. Her mother started to have mental health issues in her 60s and I strongly believe that these heavy metals had a lot to do with it. Other stressors also played a part in it, but I believe this was the strongest. We started working on this right away with my mother so she wouldn't face similar challenges. I started to do oral chelation to try to eliminate the burden of heavy metals in my body. I believe that chelation can be dangerous if done improperly so you must know what you are doing. Many medical and alternative practitioners go about this wrongly and it can be detrimental to your health so be careful if you choose to do this.

In a Forbes magazine article titled *Chelation Therapy: What To Do With Inconvenient Evidence,* Cardiologist Harlan Krumholz discusses a $31 million trial of chelation therapy by the National Institutes of Health that found very positive results from chelation therapy. He says, "The irony is that if a drug manufacturer had gotten this result, they would have celebrated. We have billion dollar drugs like niacin and fenofibrate and ezetimibe that have less evidence than chelation therapy has now. None of those drugs has contemporary outcomes studies showing benefit—and 2 of them (niacin and fenofibrate) have 2 recent negative trials."[17] He is basically saying that because chelation is not making billions of dollars for a drug company you will not hear about it.

Dr. Dan Pompa is a leader in heavy metal chelation. He struggled for years with his own illness and has tried about every method available. Here is what he says about chelation, "Let's start with the alternative side of things. Herbs are great for many things and so are homeopathic remedies, but when it comes to heavy metal chelation, they are not "true chelators." Therefore, they fail to do a good job of removing the metals completely from the body. Metals such as mercury and lead got their name "heavy" metals title for good reason; they are in fact very heavy. Due to their physical weight and some other unique properties, heavy metals can deplete the body of its natural detoxification properties such as sulfur, certain amino acids and enzymes, glutathione, and methyl groups. Once this occurs the heavy metals begin to bio-accumulate in the body and worse yet, in the brain. Heavy metals are not like other toxins; they not only eventually exhaust precious detoxification pathways, which allow the bio-accumulation of other toxins, but can in turn cause other toxicity issues from infections.

Heavy metals will allow a safe haven for pathogens such as candida and Lyme. The immune cells will not come near the toxic mercury, so the pathogens adapt and hide from the immune system around the mercury. I could never get rid of my chronic candida until I got my metal burden lowered to a certain level. The Lyme bacteria and heavy metals have a unique synergy as well. It is estimated that 90% of the population in certain parts of the country have Lyme disease; so why are they all not sick? Lyme, like other pathogens such as candida, herpes virus, Epstein Barr virus and others are opportunistic and will only affect someone who is immune compromised. This is what heavy metals like mercury do; they provide an altered terrain, which is ripe for the bad guys. Most, if not all, Lyme disease sufferers have heavy metal issues and both need to be addressed for lasting recovery.

To successfully chelate heavy metals out of the body and brain, and to prevent the dangers of re-absorption, a "true chelator" must be used. Herbs such as cilantro, or binding agents like chlorella, do not have the molecular structure to hold on to a heavy metal permanently. Therefore, they only stir up the metals and cause them to redistribute somewhere else. Most likely, they end up in the brain and cause more bizarre and unexplainable symptoms. These types of detox agents do not contain a double "SH group" called a "thiol group". I will spare you the biochemistry lecture, but it is this "double thiol group" that is able to properly bind heavy metals and safely escort them out of the body. This is in fact defines a "true chelator", and is the only safe and effective agent at the present time to remove heavy metals.

Many doctors perform IV chelation using a prescription true chelating agent such as DMPS (2,3-dimercapto-1-propanesulfonic acid), and unlike the herbals and other binders I mentioned above, it works! The problem with using IV chelation therapies is that they will pull a lot of heavy metals all at once and do not stay in the body long enough and therefore can cause redistribution of heavy metals. DMPS and DMSA are water soluble and go in and out of the body very quickly. Because it pulls heavy metals so well and yet leaves the body so quickly, it sets up a concentration gradient in the body, initiating the remaining metals to move out of the tissues. Let's go back to basic chemistry and remember that things move from higher concentration to lower concentration area in the body. The problem is the chelating agent has moved out of the body, bringing heavy metals with it. This leaves a lower concentration area behind, causing the deeper stored metals in the body to move out of the tissues into circulation, only to redistribute somewhere else. This can cause many unwanted symptoms and worse yet, if it crosses into the brain, you have made a bad situation catastrophic."[14]

I studied under Dr. Pompa and have seen the amazing results from his protocols. I started to notice a difference when I began chelating. My irritability dramatically decreased and my clarity improved immensely. Three months into chelation I passed all of the parasites that were built up in my gut. I noticed a huge improvement in my health after that. It turns out that the doctor who did my colonoscopy wasn't crazy after all. Chelation done properly will take months or even years to complete. About eleven months into chelation I actually started to feel worse again and I couldn't figure out why. I started to notice fatigue, irritability, and weight gain setting in. I was looking everywhere for the source. I had a dental cleaning appointment that same month and when I was visiting the dentist the assistant asked if I knew that I had two amalgams on the back of my molars. I had no idea they were even there, I didn't even remember having them in. Then it hit me, the chelation I was doing was pulling metal from the fillings and making me worse. I immediately scheduled to have them removed from an IAOMT certified dentist. After the removal it took me a few months to start feeling well again, but I finally did after several rounds of chelation. You can probably see why I believe you should never have chelation done if you have amalgam fillings in your mouth.

There are no long term studies that show the effect of amalgams, I'm talking 40-50 years, only short term studies. You'll have to judge for yourself whether you think they are doing you harm. There are studies that show the effects of long term use of mercury in the workplace. This study showed significantly decreased strength, decreased coordination, increased tremor, decreased sensation, and increased prevalence of Babinski and snout reflexes in people who worked with elemental mercury 20-35 years previously[11]. A Canadian Study showed double the urine mercury levels of people who had amalgams[12]. A study from the British Dental Journal found that dentist had 4 times higher mercury urine levels[13]. Does that mean we can say that it is doing harm in them just because the urine levels are higher? No, it doesn't. With mercury being one of the most toxic substances known to man you can make up your own mind on that one.

Most major countries other than the U.S. have extensive bans and health warnings regarding the use of amalgam fillings. This includes countries suchas Austria, Australia, Canada, France, Great Britain, Japan, New Zealand, Norway, Sweden, and Switzerland.

In 1988, scrap dental amalgam material was declared hazardous waste by the EPA. OSHA has certain mandates present to handle amalgam fillings before they go into and out of your mouth.

1. Scrap amalgam must be stored in an unbreakable, tight sealed container away from heat.

2. Use a no-touch technique for handling the amalgam.
3. Store under liquid, preferably glycerin or photographic fixer solution.

These are common mercury symptoms.
- Depression
- Mild fatigue
- Anxiety
- Forgetfulness
- Eyelid, face, or muscle twitching
- Digestive issues
- Constipation and or diarrhea
- Frequent bad breath
- Constant body odor
- Dizziness
- Irritability
- Sensitivity to sound
- Inability to concentrate (Brain Fog)
- Abnormal menses
- Low body temperature
- Cold hands and feet
- Tender teeth
- Tinnitus (Ringing in the ears)
- Insomnia
- Metallic taste in the mouth
- Nail fungus
- Unexplained Anger
- Autoimmune response

Many people struggle with odd or unexplainable symptoms and cannot seem to get rid of them no matter what they try. You should definitely consider looking at heavy metals. Below you can see my mother's test and my test.

To learn more about heavy metals visit
http://www.inflammationdetox.com/getfreevideos

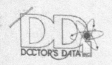

LAB #: U121115-2422-1
PATIENT: Chance Haugen
ID: HAUGEN-C-00047
SEX: Male
AGE: 28

CLIENT #: 38914
DOCTOR: Chance Haugen, DC
Big Stone Chiropractic
16 2nd St Nw
Ortonville, MN 56278 USA

Toxic Metals; Urine

TOXIC METALS

		RESULT µg/g creat	REFERENCE INTERVAL	WITHIN REFERENCE	OUTSIDE REFERENCE
Aluminum	(Al)	4.9	< 25		
Antimony	(Sb)	< dl	< 0.3		
Arsenic	(As)	12	< 108		
Barium	(Ba)	10	< 7		
Beryllium	(Be)	< dl	< 1		
Bismuth	(Bi)	< dl	< 10		
Cadmium	(Cd)	< dl	< 0.8		
Cesium	(Cs)	4.4	< 9		
Gadolinium	(Gd)	< dl	< 0.3		
Lead	(Pb)	8	< 2		
Mercury	(Hg)	4.6	< 3		
Nickel	(Ni)	1.9	< 10		
Palladium	(Pd)	< dl	< 0.3		
Platinum	(Pt)	< dl	< 1		
Tellurium	(Te)	< dl	< 0.8		
Thallium	(Tl)	0.2	< 0.5		
Thorium	(Th)	< dl	< 0.03		
Tin	(Sn)	1.3	< 9		
Tungsten	(W)	0.6	< 0.4		
Uranium	(U)	< dl	< 0.03		

URINE CREATININE

	RESULT mg/dL	REFERENCE INTERVAL	-2SD	-1SD	MEAN	+1SD	+2SD
Creatinine	57.4	45 - 225					

SPECIMEN DATA

Comments:

Date Collected:	11/13/2012	pH upon receipt: Acceptable	Collection Period: timed: 6 hours
Date Received:	11/15/2012	<dl less than detection limit	Volume:
Date Completed:	11/16/2012	Provoking Agent: DMSA	Provocation: POST PROVOCATIVE
Method:	ICP-MS	Creatinine by Jaffe Method	

Results are creatinine corrected to account for urine dilution variations. **Reference intervals and corresponding graphs are representative of a healthy population under non-provoked conditions.** Chelation (provocation) agents can increase urinary excretion of metals/elements.

V13

©DOCTOR'S DATA, INC. • ADDRESS: 3755 Illinois Avenue, St. Charles, IL 60174-2420 • CLIA ID NO: 14D0646470 • MEDICARE PROVIDER NO: 148453

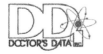

LAB #: U121025-2050-1
PATIENT: Mary Haugen
ID: HAUGEN-M-00044
SEX: Female
AGE: 53

CLIENT #: 38914
DOCTOR: Chance Haugen, DC
Big Stone Chiropractic
16 2nd St Nw
Ortonville, MN 56278 USA

Toxic Metals; Urine

TOXIC METALS		RESULT µg/g creat	REFERENCE INTERVAL	WITHIN REFERENCE	OUTSIDE REFERENCE
Aluminum	(Al)	11	< 35	▬	
Antimony	(Sb)	< dl	< 0.4		
Arsenic	(As)	20	< 117	▬	
Barium	(Ba)	1.9	< 7	▬	
Beryllium	(Be)	< dl	< 1		
Bismuth	(Bi)	< dl	< 15		
Cadmium	(Cd)	0.5	< 1	▬▬	
Cesium	(Cs)	5.2	< 10	▬▬	
Gadolinium	(Gd)	< dl	< 0.4		
Lead	(Pb)	22	< 2	▬▬▬▬▬▬▬▬▬▬▬▬▬	
Mercury	(Hg)	14	< 4	▬▬▬▬▬▬▬▬▬▬	
Nickel	(Ni)	1.7	< 12	▬	
Palladium	(Pd)	< dl	< 0.3		
Platinum	(Pt)	< dl	< 1		
Tellurium	(Te)	< dl	< 0.8		
Thallium	(Tl)	0.3	< 0.5	▬▬▬	
Thorium	(Th)	< dl	< 0.03		
Tin	(Sn)	3.9	< 10	▬▬	
Tungsten	(W)	< dl	< 0.4		
Uranium	(U)	< dl	< 0.04		

URINE CREATININE	RESULT mg/dL	REFERENCE INTERVAL	-2SD	-1SD	MEAN	+1SD	+2SD
Creatinine	42.3	35- 225		▬▬▬▬▬			

SPECIMEN DATA

Comments:

Date Collected:	10/24/2012	pH upon receipt: Acceptable	Collection Period: timed: 6 hours
Date Received:	10/25/2012	<dl: less than detection limit	Volume:
Date Completed:	10/29/2012	Provoking Agent: DMSA	Provocation: POST PROVOCATIVE
Method:	ICP-MS	Creatinine by Jaffe Method	

Results are creatinine corrected to account for urine dilution variations. **Reference intervals and corresponding graphs are representative of a healthy population under non-provoked conditions.** Chelation (provocation) agents can increase urinary excretion of metals/elements.

V13

©DOCTOR'S DATA, INC. • ADDRESS: 3755 Illinois Avenue, St. Charles, IL 60174-2420 • CLIA ID NO: 14D0646470 • MEDICARE PROVIDER NO: 148453

0001623

Chapter 11-Biotoxins

I had new windows put in my home and we were really excited about it. They looked so much better and we could definitely tell that they helped with our heating and cooling bills. After a few months passed I noticed that the paint on the bottom window sill was starting to rub off and I thought that was odd. We had a really wet spring and I was wondering if maybe water got in somehow. I looked all around the window and when I looked down by the floor at the bottom of the window I noticed that the wall had some moist black spots on it. I called up the contractor and he came over. When we looked at the window we noticed that the caulking had fallen off leaving gaps at the bottom of the window outside. He agreed that we should take the wall apart and look inside. When we opened it up there was a puddle of water and mold growing on the backside of the drywall. If we had left this problem, or not found it, it could have gotten worse and it is possible members of my family may have gotten sick. If someone had gotten sick it would have been difficult for a doctor to diagnose it is as mold illness if we didn't know there was water leaking into the home. This is why mold illness and biotoxic illness can be hard to find if you don't know what you are looking for.

According to the Occupational Safety and Health Administration, 20 million American workers—or 15% of the country's work force—are affected by toxic fungi related to sick building syndrome. It's estimated that 10 million US school kids are exposed daily to building related fungal toxins. Biotoxins are organisms that can drive inflammation in your body and the two biggest ones that we know of that do this are mold and lyme. These are probably two of the bigger health issues that are really misunderstood and misdiagnosed.

Mold illness can be tough to spot if you are not familiar with it. Dr. Richie Shoemaker, a leading researcher in mold illness, says that twenty-five percent of the country is genetically susceptible to these mold toxins. The thing that's really driving it is our new way that we build houses. We used to have more airy, drafty houses where air could get through. Today houses are so airtight that they create the perfect environment for mold. If you start to get water in a spot and no air is getting to it then you are going to have mold. Then you put things like an HVAC unit in and keep all the air inside the house. You've got the perfect climate control for your new tenant—mold.

Mold also needs things to eat like drywall and wood. Now if you include basements where it's dark, where it grows best and probably where you're more likely to get water exposure, you've got the perfect spot for mold to start growing.

The two things that will determine if you get sick are your genes and how full your bucket is. You can't control your genes, but you can control your environment and how full your bucket is. Mold illness is something that is fairly easy to overcome as long as you know that mold is the culprit. The fix, though, can sometimes be a hassle, especially if you have to fix your house or move out of your house. Convincing your employer to make changes may not be easy either.

Another bio-toxin, lyme, has been basically ignored. Just last year the CDC finally came out and said it's not 30,000 cases per year in the US, it's 300,000 cases. I actually think it's even more than that because the testing for Lyme Disease is so poor. A test like Western blot, which is what most clinicians are going to use is kind of like flipping a coin, 50/50. Let's say that you have Lyme, there is only a 50% chance that the test will say that you have it. That's how bad the test is. There are a lot of people having tests done that are sick but are showing that they're not because the testing is so poor.

There are new tests coming along like the ispot lyme test from Neuroscience that are much more accurate at testing for lyme. The problem is that these tests have not become mainstream yet.

How would you know if a bio-toxin is affecting you? Well, it can affect multiple systems in your body, also if you're having mold issues a lot of time there are other stressors going on like heavy metals and both have to be dealt with at the same time or you may not see results.

Common Bio-Toxin Symptoms

- chronic respiratory infections
- shortness of breath
- shooting pain
- sore muscles
- fibromyalgia symptoms
- extreme tightness and aches
- migratory joint pain, inflammation
- chronic fatigue
- excessive thirst
- excessive urination
- excessive sweating or body odor
- sensitivity to light and sound
- chemical sensitivities
- skin sensitivities
- skin infections
- recurring infections
- mold eyes- glazed eyes, red eyes
- brain fog
- short term memory loss
- ADHD

All of these things can actually be underlying bio-toxic illness. That's why we need to start playing better detectives when it comes to our health and not just trying to cover things up because if you have this problem going on in your home, it's going to stay there. You're going to continue to be sick or your kids are going to continue to be sick or possibly get sick.

To learn more about biotoxins visit
http://www.inflammationdetox.com/getfreevideos

Chapter 12-Electronics

"If you wish to understand the secrets of the Universe, think of energy, frequency, and vibration." Nikola Tesla

I hated physics. I didn't like all of the math and equations, not my thing. I did find it extremely interesting though, as long as I didn't have to complete an equation. One of the most interesting laws that I remember is the law of conservation of energy. Energy cannot be created or destroyed, only changed from one form into another or transferred from one object to another. This is happening constantly and we don't even realize it.

Energy, frequencies, and vibrations are everywhere, they are all around us. With each day new technologies are released that put us around more of these unseen wonders. Even though you can't see them, it doesn't mean they aren't having a profound impact on your health. Energy can help our health or it can have a very negative impact.

Radiation is one that we know we should be avoiding. Don't sit with your laptop on your lap frying your reproductive organs and try to keep your cell phone out of your pocket. Use a Bluetooth headset if you have to be on your cell phone for a long period of time.

An emerging area of concern is with EMF's or electromagnetic frequencies. EMF's are low energy frequencies emitted from all kinds of electronic devices. Studies suggesting that they can interfere with some of our biological processes are mounting. One of the biggest areas where it can disturb your health is in your sleep cycle. If you are having trouble sleeping make sure you don't have your cell phone or computer next to the bed. Your router shouldn't be in your bed room either. Maybe you live under power lines or next to a cell tower. These are all things that could potentially be affecting your health. If you are struggling with health issues it is always best to take as much burden off your body as possible. Limiting your exposure to EMF's may help.

Chapter 13-Emotional Health

I want you to do something for me. I want to show you how powerful a thought is in your body, what it does, and how your thinking plays such a huge role in your health.

Now what I want you to do is imagine that someone just came up and told you that someone close to you has passed away. What do you start to feel? You can start to feel your body change, right? You start to feel your heartbeat increase; your blood pressure rises as anxiety and depression set in; your mind begins to race; tears may start to come. All of these things are hormonal changes taking place in the body from one single thought.

If you stay in a state like this for a long period of time, what happens? It's not healthy, is it? Your body starts to use stress hormones to deal with the situation. You begin to deplete methyl groups and vital nutrients in your body and this drives inflammation. If this state becomes chronic it will lead to a disease. You can see how just from one single thought, inflammation can begin to drive disease throughout your body.

This is how powerful our thoughts and emotions are in our body. We have to learn how to control what we're thinking and what we're feeling. I'm not saying that responding to a situation like that is bad. What I'm saying is when you're under that kind of stress and having that kind of thought all the time, that's when it's bad. And so we literally have to start to think differently. You have to start to mold what you want it to be and who you want to be. You have to consciously start to work at this.

To show you how stress can age you take a look at President Obama. Compare pictures of him right before his presidency with pictures taken right now. Quite a difference. I'm sure there is a tiny bit of pressure that comes with being the President of the United States.

When you get up in the morning, one of the first things that you have to do is control your thoughts. Most of you have heard about this and considered it, but have never taken the time to do it. Whether you do this through daily affirmations or through reading scripture, you need to start. It's going to slowly start to change how you think and how you feel about yourself. When you start to think differently you will see that not only will you handle stress better, but you are going to treat other people better and your relationships will get better.

You also have to believe and be thankful for where you're at in your life. Because where you are is great, and you're meant to be where you're at for a reason. Almost everyone who is reading this wants their life to be different in some way, or thinks that their life could be better, or they want somebody else's life. It's sad but we all do it. You need to stop doing it and be grateful; what you have right now is great. You need to realize that. It's great to have goals and strive to achieve them, but at the same time you need to enjoy what you have been given.

Start to enjoy the moments that you are in everyday. Don't let TV, cell phones, and the internet steal them from you. Don't live through other people on TV shows and social media, get out and do your own thing.

Unhappy people do many of the following things I'm going to list below. Take these belief systems and switch them around. I'm not saying it will come easy, but if you make an effort with them you will start to see change in your life.

If you relate to one of these then make an effort to change.

- You Believe Most People Can't Be Trusted
- You Believe Life Is Hard
- You Compare Yourself to Others Too Often
- You Concentrate On What Is Wrong With the World
- You Gossip and Complain
- You Strive To Control Everything
- You Worry About Every Detail

Be Grateful. Wake up every morning thankful, and go out with intention to impact somebody's life in a positive way. Any time you do something nice for someone, how do you feel? It usually makes you feel pretty good, right? So when we start to live for other people instead of ourselves and our selfish interest it will actually benefit us more. It's amazing how it works, but the more you focus on helping other people the more it is going to help you.

If you make an effort to start to do that, it becomes a habit. I guarantee it will have a positive effect on your life and your emotional health, and this is going to be a stressor that you can eliminate.

Chapter 14-Physical Stressors

There are many physical stressors and I'm sure you are aware of many of them in your life. I want to talk about one that you probably are not aware of. When my son was born one of his shoulders got hung up on the way out and we had to rotate his shoulders and arms to get him out. When he came out he was having a little trouble breathing. I immediately checked the area we had to twist slightly to get him out and I adjusted his 1st cervical vertebrae and his first thoracic vertebrae. His breathing immediately went back to normal. The midwife was amazed at the quick recovery. Most kids don't have the luxury of getting adjusted right after birth because the parents are unaware of the connection between birth trauma and health issues.

Some degree of spinal birth trauma happens in over 80% of births. It is easy to see how this can happen and it is hard to avoid, even in natural births. Watch a few births, especially C-sections on YouTube and you can see how spinal trauma can occur. Dr. Tony Ebel is a leader in birth trauma and his teaching is helping us look at childhood health problems in new way.[16] With all the pulling and rotating it is easy to have a misalignment happen. This misalignment then becomes fixated or stuck and this leads to nervous system disruption. You live your life through your nervous system. Your nervous system is what connects your brain to every other part of your body and as soon as you start to disrupt it your body cannot communicate properly with itself. The wrong signals are sent and disease processes start in your body. Muscles are also affected in the neck and head region. They become tight and don't allow fluid to drain out of the ears. Most pediatricians will tell you that kids have more ear infections because gravity cannot help push fluid out the ears because their Eustachian tubes are more horizontal than those of adults. This is only partially true. They are more horizontal, but motion drains the ears more than gravity. When everything in the neck and head becomes fixated it becomes impossible for motion to help drain the ears and you get ear infections. This is why chiropractic adjustments are the most effective remedy for ear infections and why antibiotics almost never work long term. If you don't fix the cause of the problem they will continue to occur. With the fixation and nervous system interruption it also leaves the kids more vulnerable to getting sick because their immune system can be compromised.

You can almost predict the path of kids who have reoccuring ear infections because they never resolve the cause of the problem. After antibiotics don't work they will have tubes put in; this will relieve the pressure in the ears, but it forces the problem further down the road. Pretty soon you'll have swollen adenoids and tonsils and strep infections. Antibiotics to the rescue, but infections will continue to happen and so you better have the tonsils and adenoids out because you're told they are the cause of the problem. You can guess what happens next, now we have forced the fluid further south and we start to see asthma and allergies because the lungs are now getting all of that drainage.

Trauma can also stimulate NMDA receptors in the brain and trigger the NO/ONOO cycle. Dr. Martin Pall is the leading expert with the NO/ONOO cycle. He believes the NO/ONOO cycle is the reason for so many unexplainable illnesses.[15] NMDA receptors are excitatory to the body and can put kids into a fight or flight response. Their bodies get stuck in sympathetic mode and they can't hit their brake pedal and relax. This explains things like colic and many ADHD symptoms. They just constantly go, go, go, because their nervous system is stuck in that state. Now after all the antibiotics, surgeries, inhalers, medications, and bad diets we have sick kids who are now stuck in a sick care system.

I use this example as a physical stressor because it is the most overlooked area in our society and it makes the absolute biggest difference between a life of happiness and a life of sickness and suffering.

Physical stressors must be addressed in your life because they can be affecting you in ways that you don't even realize.

Chapter 15-Exercise

When I was dealing with all of my health issues I was still exercising because I was trying so desperately to lose weight. When I was done exercising though it felt like I was burnt out and had no energy, that isn't the way I used to feel. Before I was sick I always felt a lot better after exercise. When your body is dealing with a lot of stressors I believe that exercise can be detrimental to your health. Your body needs to focus on fixing a few things before you try to become the next Hulk Hogan otherwise you can actually drive inflammation in your body.

Now I'm not saying that exercise is bad; the right kind of exercise is great for the body. Once you have the proper nutrition protocols in place and have decreased inflammation throughout your body you should do great with exercise.

I enjoy watching the Olympics and there is something I want you to pay attention to the next time you watch the summer Olympics. Compare long distance runners to sprinters. You're going to notice a huge difference in their physique. Sprinters are ripped and muscular while the long distance runners are what I call skinny fat. The reason why is because of the type of hormones they are training their bodies to release during exercise.

The most beneficial type of exercise is high intensity or burst training, which is very similar to sprinting. This type of exercise increases your heart rate for a short period of time, usually 30-60 seconds. Then you allow the heart rate to drop to normal and you repeat this cycle about five to seven times.

This type of training puts you into a fight or flight response while you train. You begin to burn sugar immediately for energy and then for the next 2 days your body will burn fat to restore energy. You start to burn more fat with this type of exercise as the growth hormone, testosterone, and other fat burning hormones are released. They are anabolic hormones that are only released during high intensity training. It also helps you become more hormone sensitive to insulin and leptin, the two major players with blood sugar and fat storage.

The opposite effect occurs with low intensity exercise. You burn fat during the workout, that is why they try to keep you in the "fat burning zone", and you burn sugar afterward. I would much rather burn fat for 2 days than for 30-60 minutes.

Chapter 16-Degenerative Diseases

I-Heart Health

Degenerative diseases are what many Americans are struggling with every single day and we need to get to the root cause. One of the most important degenerative diseases to me is heart disease just because of the huge impact it's had on my family. I've lost loved ones to heart disease, heart attacks, and strokes just like most of you have. If we are going to stop these terrible diseases we need to start thinking differently.

I believe that the number one reason for heart disease is actually inflammation. Americans are told that cholesterol is the cause of heart disease and I believe that is very misleading. Cholesterol causes inflammation when it becomes oxidized. To understand oxidation better I want you to think of rust. Oxidation in your blood vessels is similar to rust on your car. When cholesterol becomes oxidized it can then increase plaque in the arteries, but the cholesterol isn't there to cause plaque it is there to do its job. Cholesterol is deployed in the bloodstream to help repair damage to your blood vessels. When you artificially lower cholesterol you may reduce oxidized cholesterol some, but you prevent cholesterol from fixing the underlying problem which allows the inflammation of the blood vessel to continue. This is why 50% of people who have heart attacks have normal cholesterol levels. It would seem like a better idea to stop doing the things that are damaging your blood vessels in the first place, and then cholesterol would stop becoming oxidized.

Cholesterol is essential for life because no cell can be made without it. Cholesterol is essential for your cell membranes, hormones, vitamin D synthesization, and so many other processes. This is why lowering cholesterol too much increases a person's risk of dying.

Cholesterol also carries out essential functions within your cell membranes, and is critical for proper brain function and production of steroid hormones, including your sex hormones. Vitamin D is also synthesized from a close relative of cholesterol: 7-dehydrocholesterol. Your body is composed of trillions of cells that need to interact with each other. Cholesterol is one of the molecules that allow for these interactions to take place.

If you want to learn more about cholesterol and the role it has in the body you can watch our free video series here:
http://www.inflammationdetox.com/getfreevideos

II-Arthritis

My dad is in his mid-50s and about 10 years ago he started to develop pain in his thumbs. He called it arthritis and just dealt with the pain. The pain didn't start very bad, but progressed over the next few years. I've had my dad address many of the points that I talk about in the book because I didn't want to have to deal with the burden that I've seen my parents go through with their parents when their health fell apart. Kind of selfish I know, but I want them around for a while and I want them to be healthy and not just laying around in a nursing home bed for 15 years waiting to die. We may have an average lifespan of about 80 years in this country, but if I live that long I want it to be a quality life. I don't want to be sitting in a home somewhere just breathing; I'd rather be with my creator if that were the case. My dad called me last fall while he was in the field to thank me because he realized that he hadn't had any joint pain in his thumbs for months. Arthritis is inflammation of the joint and if you can get the inflammation to stop a lot of the time the joint pain will go away. I'm not saying that you can reverse the damage that has been done, but I am saying that if you can get the inflammatory process to stop most of the time the pain will stop and this is what happened in my dad's case. The two biggest changes that he made that stopped this process were his dietary changes and the chelation therapy that he went through.

III-Hormones

If you ask women when their problems started, a lot of them will say it was after a pregnancy. I believe that is because they go through so many hormone and body changes that it allows toxins to be released from the body. The musculoskeletal changes and the hormonal changes become stressors in women who are toxic and this leads their bucket to overflow. Genes can be turned on and off from those stressors and now many health issues begin after the pregnancy.

Suzanne Somers attributed a 24 urine hormone test to saving her life. It allowed her to look at different estrogen levels in her body. Some estrogens become toxic in the body and can lead to cancer. One of the biggest reasons that allow these estrogens to become dominant is lack of methyl groups in the body. I described methylation earlier in the book and this is why it is so important. Methyl groups attach to toxic estrogen and this helps the body remove it. If there are other stressors going on in a woman's life and methyl groups are depleted you can begin to have hormonal issues. You can take certain supplements to help increase methyl groups in the body, but the main thing you want to do is get rid of the stressors depleting them in your body.

> If you want to learn more about hormones and methylation you can watch our free video series here.
> http://www.inflammationdetox.com/getfreevideos

IV-Blood Sugar

Diabetes is rarely a cause of death. It's usually some other degenerative disease such as heart disease or stroke. Why do diabetics struggle with so many other degenerative diseases? Because they're so inflamed from high blood glucose levels that insulin is not heard by the cell and then this leads to other inflammatory issues. We all know that diet and exercise will help diabetics manage the disease better, but what role can reducing toxins play?

They now say that 30% of diabetes could be from toxin issues. We know that smoking can cause diabetes. Why is that? Because of the toxins from the smoke. What about all the other toxins in our lives, can they lead to diabetes? Absolutely and I think that this is going to be something that you're going to see addressed more in the years to come. We will hopefully start to look at this more as a cause of diabetes. 29.1 million Americans—or 9.3% of the population—have diabetes and most have never thought of it as a toxin issue. Eliminate grains and sugars from your diet and start to detox and more than likely you will see positive results with your blood sugar!

V-Thyroid

The American Association of Clinical Endocrinologists estimate that 27 million people suffer from thyroid disease in the US or have a thyroid issue. Most women won't test positive for thyroid disease for 10 to 20 years. It's estimated that 80% of women over the age of 40 have sub optimal thyroid function.

Blood tests for thyroid may not be accurate or the right blood tests may even be skipped. Normal blood test values are determined by a healthy population of people, but if the majority is suffering from thyroid problems then you can imagine what that will do to the blood test values. It increases them greatly. We have our coaching clients consider using different values when they get their results back. I believe these values are more of an optimal range and most thyroid experts would agree.

If you dig deeper into thyroid issues, it's estimated that 80% of women who have hypothyroid problems are autoimmune. Most women don't even know if they're autoimmune because the tests have never been run. The reason why I think that this test isn't run is because there's nobody pushing it because there's no medication for it if it does come back abnormal. There's really no medical solution for this issue. I believe that if you take the principles that we're teaching in this book and apply them, you might see some results on your own. You have to know what you're dealing with first and so getting these right tests is absolutely imperative.

If you want to learn more about your thyroid then follow this link and watch our free video series.
http://www.inflammationdetox.com/getfreevideos

Chapter 17-Value

One of the biggest hurdles or things that will stop people from making changes in their life is money. The fact of the matter is that if you don't pay for something you don't value it and you won't follow through with it. The one thing that I have found out is that if I have something that is important to me or something that I want to accomplish I want to pay for it or I will never do it or follow through with it. If you had free gym membership would you go as often as one that you paid for? I know I wouldn't. In our society; if we don't pay for something we quit it or stop using it. If a goal is important to you invest in it and you will have a much better chance of succeeding. Everyone should be investing in their health; unfortunately most of us are just reactive instead of proactive. We will pay for something once it is broken or once it is has gotten to the point that we can no longer stand it. The problem with this is that in this country it is going to cost you a lot of money if you get sick. Insurance rates, hospital bills, medications, and large deductibles have us spending a lot of money of health care that we could be using elsewhere.

In 2012 the average person spent $8,915 on health care. With health care premiums jumping the last couple of years, I'm sure this number has gone up. Chronic disease accounts for $3 of every $4 spent on health care. Most of those diseases are preventable. According to a report published in *The Journal of General Internal Medicine*; 25% of older adults incurred out of pocket medical expenses that exceeded the total value of their assets. 43% incurred expenses that exceeded their assets, excluding the value of their home.

People with Alzheimer's spent on average $66,155 during the last five years of their life; cancer patients spent $32,129; cardiovascular patients spent $37,996; diabetic patients spent $38,517. Those are just the last five years of their life. There were more than likely significant amounts spent on health issues before the last five years as well. According to Afflac, the average out of pocket expense for a heart attack is $5,000-$8000. The average for a stroke is $23,380. Colon cancer is $15,000-$17,000. Lung cancer care is between $323-$8,011 per month. Breast cancer is $712 a month. Type 2 diabetics incurs on average $11,744 per year of out of pocket expenses.

It will cost you a lot if you allow yourself to develop a chronic disease. You don't have to waste your hard earned life savings on your health. Start making changes now and stop all this madness. Little investments now like food, gym memberships, and health coaching can save you big amounts later. Whatever area it is that you need to work on, if you spend money on it you will have better results. Always remember that when you are trying to accomplish something in your life.

Chapter 18-Hope

I want to leave you with hope. There are answers out there and controlling inflammation in your body can have huge health benefits. I hope you'll consider the information in this book even if it is something you haven't thought of before or even if you find it odd or unusual. When your health problems start to snowball, it gets hard. It can be difficult to dig through everything and find the causes. I've been there. The question is are you willing to do the things that are necessary and are you willing to put in the time and effort to get well, because I'm not going to tell you that it is a walk in the park, but it is definitely achievable. There is no magic cure or magic pill.

The biggest issue that I see with most people is that they think that an answer's going to come overnight—it's going to take a month, it's going to take two months—and that's not so. This has taken years to build. It's been in and around your life for a long time more than likely, and in no way can you expect your body to completely transform overnight. It's going to take time, it's going to take energy, and it's going to take some work, but it can be done. I don't want to make it sound like it's impossible to achieve, but I want you to know it won't be handed to you. The hardest part is breaking old habits and replacing them with good, healthy habits.

What does healthy mean to you? Does it mean that just because you don't have symptoms you are healthy or can you be unhealthy and not have symptoms? I hope after all of this you can see how your bucket can be filling with no outward symptoms.

Imagine your life 1 year from now with no changes—5 years from now—the prescriptions, surgeries, body aches, depression, low energy, weight gain, hormones. Don't accept this. Start implementing change in your life and make it how you want it and 5 years from now you will be amazed at the positive impact it has had on your life.

Chapter 19-The Inflammation Detox

Now that you've seen the biggest factors that are driving inflammation in your life, I would like to invite you to watch several videos that will introduce you to the opportunity of using a system that will help you quickly and efficiently eliminate inflammation from your life.

These videos will reveal a step-by-step process for finding toxins in your life, inspiring case studies of other people who have already gone through the process.

Follow the link to learn more.

http://www.inflammationdetox.com/getfreevideos

Chapter 20-Success Stories

We've seen a lot of people have huge breakthroughs after decreasing inflammation in their body. I'd like to share a few of those successes with you so you can see just how big of an impact this can have on your life. None of these testimonies are me stating that I can cure or reverse a disease, they are just what other people have experienced with decreasing inflammation in their body. I hope that your testimony is one that we can one day share.

I was struggling immensely with my thyroid when I met Dr. Chance. I had seen every specialist you can imagine and I wasn't getting any better. I was on thyroid hormone and I was still struggling with extreme fatigue, exhaustion, pain, weight loss resistance, and hair loss. Dr. Chance explained that I had not had the right tests run and when we ran the right one we found out that I was autoimmune. Once we knew I was autoimmune we began to focus on my immune system and lowering inflammation in my body. The results were spectacular and I feel like a completely different person.
Nancy

I was overweight and I knew it was starting to affect my health negatively. I had back pain, knee pain, and some nerve issues in my feet. I struggled with self control and needed a way to make better habits. Dr. Chance helped explain what exactly is healthy and what is not. He helped make it easy for me while I was on the road so I wouldn't eat unhealthy fast food. His ideas on how to make new habits and making healthy substitutions work great. I've lost 60 pounds and my pains are gone.
Tony

When I first met Dr. Chance I was overweight and on anxiety and depression medications. I couldn't lose weight no matter what diet I tried. Dr. Chance showed me how inflammation was affecting my weight loss hormones and gave me the tools I needed to address it. I've now lost 60 pounds and my physician took me off of all my medications.
Lori

I was struggling with my blood sugar and medications were not lowering it. I was on several other medications for other problems. I had neuropathy in my feet and a diabetic microaneurysm in my eye. After using Dr. Chance's advice my regular physician was able to take me off all my medications. My blood sugar is controlled with just my diet. My neuropathy is gone and my microaneurysm is gone. My husband was also able to get off his cholesterol medication and blood pressure medication. He is a trucker and now knows how to stay healthy when he is on the road. I can't thank Dr. Chance enough for helping my husband and I completely change our lives.
Beth

Tom lost 65lbs.

Danny lost 80lbs.

Bonnie lost 65lbs.

Sandy's M.D. told her she no longer needs her diabetic medication after just 2 months. She is saving over $150 a month in prescription refills.

Judy has had to change her eye glass prescription because her eyes continue to get better and better.

Before I started care there were many foods I couldn't eat including the majority of fruits and vegetables. I was told by my doctor to just avoid these foods. Dr. Chance's cultured whey gut protocol I am now eating foods that I haven't had in years! My energy level has skyrocketed!
Heather

I have been an Herbalife Distributor for 8 years; I have been struggling with my weight and was unable to lose the weight I knew I needed to lose. My blood pressure was in the high range and I was told I should be on medication. I told my doctor to give me 6 months to make it right myself, naturally, vs. medication. After completing this program I am feeling incredible!! I have great energy, I am sleeping like a baby, my skin feels amazing, my blood pressure is now in the perfect range and the

best part is I have lost a total of 26 pounds in 3 months and I am still losing. I don't classify this as a diet; really, it is just about choices and eating healthy.
Denise

Rachel tried everything to lose weight and could never lose more than 5 lbs. She has now lost over 40lbs. She states that her mood and emotions were one of the first things to improve and because of that her family life was much better.

Leon was told his kidneys were leaking protein and failing. They wanted him to start immune suppressing drugs and anti-inflammatories immediately. They also told him dialysis was in his future and possibly a transplant. I informed him I did not know If I could help, but we could certainly try. 2 months into the program his protein leaking stopped and his kidneys have returned to normal. His doctors were baffled by the change, but told him to continue what he was doing.

In one month I have regained all of the feeling in my leg that had been numb for 2 years. My glucose is under 100. I am off of my Januvia and have lowered my insulin 10 units. I've lost 10 lbs.
Kim

I was having severe gut issues. The pain and fatigue were so bad I was wondering if I would be able to continue working. I tried everything conventional medicine had for me and I was still suffering. There were so many foods I could not eat without severe pain and diarrhea. I heard Dr. Haugen speak and it was the first time that I had hope in years. I implemented what he taught me and I began to see results almost immediately. My energy began to return, the pain left, and with that the hope grew that I might lead a normal life once again. Over time I was able to start introducing foods that would have instantly made me sick before. I'm very grateful for what Dr. Haugen taught me; it has allowed me to start living again.
Robert

References

1. Dariush Mozaffarian, Haiming Cao, Irena B. King, Rozenn N. Lemaitre, Xiaoling Song, David S. Siscovick, and Gökhan S. Hotamisligil Trans-Palmitoleic Acid, Metabolic Risk Factors, and New-Onset Diabetes in U.S. Adults Annals of Internal Medicine 2010 December Harvard School of Public Health
2. Salmerón J, Hu FB, Manson JE, et al. Dietary fat intake and risk of type 2 diabetes in women. Am J Clin Nutr 2001;73:1019–26
3. Kuller (1993) Trans Fatty Acids and Dieting, The Lancet 341:1093-1094.
4. Volek JS et al. Body composition and hormonal responses to a carbohydrate-restricted diet. Metabolism. 2002 Jul;51(7):864-70. http://pmid.us/12077732
5. Danforth E Jr et al. Dietary-induced alterations in thyroid hormone metabolism during overnutrition. J Clin Invest. 1979 Nov;64(5):1336-47. http://pmid.us/500814
6. Mitchell HH, Glickman N, et al. The tolerance of man to cold as affected by dietary modification; proteins versus carbohydrate and the effect of variable protective clothing. Am J Physiol. 1946 Apr;146:66-83.
7. Wagner M, Schlüsener MP, Ternes TA, Oehlmann J (2013) Identification of Putative Steroid Receptor Antagonists in Bottled Water: Combining Bioassays and High-Resolution Mass Spectrometry. PLoS ONE 8(8): e72472. doi:10.1371/journal.pone.0072472
8. Multiple adverse thyroid and metabolic health signs in the population from the area heavily polluted by organochlorine cocktail (PCB, DDE, HCB, dioxin)
9. Pavel Langer, Anton Kočan, Mária Tajtáková, Katarína Sušienková, Žofia Rádiková, Juraj Koška, Lucia Kšinantová, Richard Imrich, Miloslava Hučková, Beáta Drobná, Daniela Gašperíková, Tomáš Trnovec, Iwar Klimeš Thyroid Res. 2009; 2: 3. Published online 2009 March 31. doi: 10.1186/1756-6614-2-3

10. Mozaffarian D, Rimm EB, Herrington DM. Dietary fats, carbohydrate, and progression of coronary atherosclerosis in postmenopausal.
11. Albers JW, Kallenbach LR, Fine LJ, Langolf GD, Wolfe RA,Donofrio PD, et al. 1988. Neurological abnormalities associated with remote occupational mercury exposure. Ann Neurol 24:651–659.
12. Zwicker JD, Dutton DJ, Emery JCH. Longitudinal analysis of the association between removal of dental amalgam, urine mercury and 14 self-reported health symptoms. Environmental Health 2014;13(1):95. doi:10.1186/1476-069X-13-95.
13. Ritchie KA, Macdonald EB, Hammersley R, O'Neil JM,McGowan DA, Dale IM, et al. 1995. A pilot study of theeffect of low level exposure to mercury on the health ofdental surgeons. Occup Environ Med 52:813–817.
14. Pompa, Daniel. "Heavy Metal Detox Done Right: Safe Heavy Metal Chelation and Mercury Amalgam Removal (When Detox Is Dangerous – Part 2 of 3)." Dr Pompa. N.p., 6 Jan. 2014. Web. 26 Jan. 2015.
15. Explaining Unexplained Ilnesses Martin L. Pall Informa Healthcare (2007)
16. Ebel, Anthony. "Ears, Antibiotics, and Asthma...Yet Another Perfect Storm | Premier Wellness Chiropractic." Premier Wellness Chiropractic. N.p., 26 Sept. 2014. Web. 26 Jan. 2015.
17. Krumholz, Harlan. "Chelation Therapy: What To Do With Inconvenient Evidence."Forbes. Forbes Magazine, 27 Mar. 2013. Web. 26 Jan. 2015.

Healthy, Fit, and Energetic

Have you been struggling with life altering fatigue, weight loss resistance, digestive issues, not sleeping well, dry skin, depression, anxiety, or trouble remembering? Have you tried diets, cutting calories, exercise, detoxes, medications and supplements with little to no success? Maybe you've lost hope and just given up. In this revolutionary new book, Chance Haugen takes your hand and leads you step-by-step through the same process he used and has used with hundreds of patients to eliminate inflammation from the body.

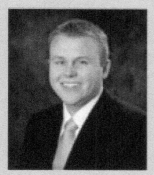 Chance had to find ways to overcome many health challenges in his own life. He went to the medical specialists and despite their best efforts he still remained sick. The health issues were starting to interfere with his career as a chiropractor and he knew he couldn't continue adjusting if things did not change. After years of struggling with digestive issues, candida, fatigue, and weight loss resistance he decided it was time to try alternative therapies. He searched and found the best alternative doctors in the country and learned directly from them. His health slowly started to improve and he got his life back. Chance then took everything he learned and utilized it to help hundreds of people get their health back. He insists that people find the true root cause of their health issues so they don't use supplements and medications to mask the real problem. He is an expert at finding what is driving inflammation and helping you eliminate it.

FOR ACCESS TO FREE
TRAINING VIDEOS PLEASE VISIT:
WWW.INFLAMMATIONDETOX.COM/GETFREEVIDEOS

Made in the USA
Coppell, TX
29 October 2021

64847581R20046